Runner's Cookbook: 10 Healthy, Tasty, and Easy to Make Recipes For Runners

All rights Reserved. No part of this publication or the information in it may be quoted from or reproduced in any form by means such as printing, scanning, photocopying or otherwise without prior written permission of the copyright holder.

Disclaimer and Terms of Use: Effort has been made to ensure that the information in this book is accurate and complete, however, the author and the publisher do not warrant the accuracy of the information, text and graphics contained within the book due to the rapidly changing nature of science, research, known and unknown facts and internet. The Author and the publisher do not hold any responsibility for errors, omissions or contrary interpretation of the subject matter herein. This book is presented solely for motivational and informational purposes only.

Table of Contents

Introduction 4

General Dietary Requirements For Runners 5

Sequential Types Of Food For Runners 7

Long Distance Runners 9

Foods For Runners 12

Whole Grain- Barley And Lentil Salad With Goat Cheese 14

Omelet Recipe For Dinner 17

Recipe For Black Beans 20

Recipes Utilizing Canned Salmon- Salmon Tacos 23

Sweet Potato Casserole Recipe 25

Strawberry Smoothie Recipe 27

Banana Smoothie Recipe 29

Peanut Butter, Banana With Chia Seed Recipe 31

Carrot- Pineapple Recipe 33

Fish With Quinoa Recipe 35

Introduction

After a very tiresome exercise of working for a very long time, there is an urge from the body that you deserve a nice treat. This is what people focus on after working very hard to earn a living. Is this similar to the athletes? What about the short distance runners do they have something in common? This is what we try to explain basing on the kind of diet these athletes ought to have before running, after running and as they relax. To them running is their day to day work and require a specific type of food.

Let us just focus on the general principles of running. The type of nutrients that gets depleted, and the kind of food is mostly utilized during the exercise. Like any other task, endurance is a virtue that most of the runners have learned to have. They spend most of their time training and finding better ways of coping with the kind of hardships that they encounter out there in the field. A lot of people would love to argue that it is a talent and not hard work. But the truth of the matter is that whether it is talent or hard work, one thing to remain, they all require a good diet.

1. Carbohydrate

There is one thing that can happen to everybody irrespective of the profession one is in. You can run out of energy if you do not take your aim to replenish that little that is remaining. For all runners after they have trained and are used to run, they both know the importance of having enough energy to keep them through the running session. If they are to compare the human body with an automobile, then the carbohydrates would be the fuel tank that can run dry if not replenished.

If you take your time and talk of most of the athletes out there on one of their worst fears when running, most of them would tell you that they fear hitting a wall. The figurative language used here implies that they are afraid of running out of energy. This occurs mostly when the amount of carbohydrates in the body gets very low and the muscles that consume this large amount of energy in the form of glucose reduces its rate of activity. The brain will definitely detect this kind of situation and send a signal to the muscles that renders it out of action.

The only way one can avoid such a scenario is to take foods that are rich in carbohydrates to keep enough energy for running.

2. Proteins

Proteins are commonly referred to as body building food. This is because they are responsible for repairing worn out tissues, muscles and many other organs. It is therefore important for an athlete to take some amount of proteins after running since most of the muscles will be worn out. The best types of proteins are those derived from cheese, white meats and eggs.

Sequential Types Of Food For Runners

Like most of the other exercise, there are those types of food that one is required to take prior to the real tasks. There is need for the athletes to balance the diets that the take during the training period, just before the event and after the event. When these balances are not observed then one could be in for a shock as most of the other competitors will be much ahead with the right gear to start the race with.

While Training

For one to be fully prepared, then you need to observe the diet a few weeks before the competition. You need to keep trying on the different types of food that can provide you with the energy you require a bit early lest you have a bad stomach during the event itself.

Since this is the preparatory stage, then you need to pay more attention to the food that release energy slowly and stores more. This will definitely call for the foods that have low GI carbohydrates as they have been found to be good at releasing energy slowly. With this, a runner will be much sure that the carbohydrate tan is fully packed waiting the right day for energy discharge. The types of food that one can take are the wholegrain rice together with the pasta.

One week prior to the real event, you will need to adjust the diet to accommodate the carbs that release energy faster. You will need to have a close relationship with food such as porridge and pasta.

Before

If you are in the long runs, then you need to take meals that have high amounts of low GI carbs before the race. The meal should also have some low amounts of proteins with some low fats as this will give you a balanced diet that will see you get through the race successfully. Some of the most common types of food that is recommended are porridge accompanied by fruits, peanut butter with bagel and many more.

During

While running the amount of carbs in the body will slowly get depleted. It has been scientifically shown that the body can only store about 2,000 kilo calories of energy. This implies that it they can only last for a few hours when you are running. Thus, after a few hours of running you will start to feel that you are week unless you replenish the energy. This therefore calls for another type of food different from those that you take while preparing because here you need fast energy.

The most recommended type of foods at this time is the high GI carbs because they release energy much faster. You can get that from food supplements such as honey, bananas and oranges. It is advisable that you get the fruits and drinks that are recommended for runners. Do not forget to take food and drinks that will keep your body fully hydrated throughout the exercise.

After

After the race, then you can stay for about 30 minutes before embarking on replenishing the body with carbs and proteins to increase the levels of energy and to repair the body muscles.

You may need to try food such as the chocolate milk combined with carbs. You are also advised to take a lot of water to replace that which is lost during while running. If you do not do this then you will probably find yourself feeling exhausted for the most part of the day afterwards.

For any runner, diet should go beyond the simple aim of maintaining a good health and incapacity the strength that he requires to perform well. The type of food they need, the way of making them and the ingredients that make the food should be carefully chosen to meet the requirements of an athlete. No wonder most of the athletes have their own chefs who see to it that they always get the best food that has been carefully vetted to be fit for every runner to win a championship keeping all other factors constant.

Some of the factors that should be kept constant are those dealing with the training, the talent and the hard work that comes solely from the runner's dedication.

1. Whole Grain Pasta And Bread

As you read this article you may be asking yourself one big question: why does a runner need such a meal? To shed light on such a question, let us go back to one of the major essential nutrient that every runner requires. The food above is rich in carbohydrates. Most of the runners need the carbohydrate to generate the energy that they need while running. Some people would argue out that if one compares the bread and the whole grain there is a significance difference among them. Bread is more processed as compared to the whole grain pasta. But even though this is the case, there is a bigger advantage that one can derive from the whole grain. Being very natural and less processed the runner gets the chance to enjoy the nutrients that come from the grain naturally.

One can also see and appreciate the advantage that the whole grains plays by imagining the rate at which runners get hungry, especially those who do long races. With the grains, the runner may not be able to feel the hunger because of the high fiber content that the grains have. This implies that most of the runners would not feel hungry while running making them perform much faster than those who take less fiber.

How To Incorporate In The Diet

You need to have a constant supply of whole grain breads, cereal together with pastas. One note that you should always remember is avoiding the white bread. This is not the only related product that you should shun as there are other products that are baked made from the white flour. All this should be avoided.

Whole Grain- Barley And Lentil Salad With Goat Cheese

Ingredients

- ¾ glass of barley

- 3 tablespoons of olive oil

- 2 tablespoons of lemon juice

- Salt and pepper

- 1 lettuce

- 1 15 ounce can lentils that is rinsed

- 1 large carrot

- ¼ red onion

- ¼ glass olives

- ¼ glass of cucumber

- 2 ounces of goat cheese

Preparation Procedures

Cook the barley following the stipulated guidelines showed in the package. As that is in progress, mix the oil with the juice and half teaspoon of salt and pepper. Mix the lettuce with ½ lemon dressing. Then mix the barley and the lentils together with the carrots, onions, olives and the cucumber together. Serve the lentils over the lettuce and then be careful to sprinkle the goat cheese as well.

2. Eggs

Research shows that one egg is capable of providing you with a tenth of all the proteins that your body requires in a given day. This can be very important to a runner who requires the proteins to rebuild the muscle tissues that may be damaged or worn out after the running sessions, the exercise and the training. This can be from the egg that each runner ought to consume to get the necessary amino acids from the egg proteins.

In addition to the proteins that a runner can get from the egg, the runner can also get the vitamin K nutrient. This is one of the most important nutrients for everyone who dreams of having healthy bones to keep him or her fit for running and participating in other sporty activities.

How To Incorporate In The Diet

There are many various ways of making eggs. Some people like them boiled, others may enjoy taking them in the form of an omelet while others will love to have them when they are poached. There are those that love them when they are fried. On most occasions, most of these methods make the consumption of an egg easy at any given time of the day.

But for an athlete, who needs to have it incorporated into a meal, then you would be required to take it for dinner or any other meal hence omelets would be more ideal.

Ingredients

- 4 eggs

- ¼ glass of milk

- 1/8 tablespoon of salt

- Pepper

- 1 tablespoon of butter

- ½ cup of chopped mushrooms

- ½ cup of chopped tomatoes

- 3 tablespoons of green onions (minced)

- ½ glass of cut Havarti cheese

Preparation Procedure

In a bowl, mix the eggs, milk, salt and the pepper. Then pour the mixture into the skillet with melted butter. With the low temperature cook the eggs. Be careful to get the eggs to the centre of the pan by pulling them using a spatula. This is done while lifting the cooked portion until they mix well.

Cook them until the eggs remain shiny and set. You can then add the vegetables together with the cheese over them. Then fold the omelets using the spatula. Cover them and cook for about one minute for the cheese to melt.

3. Beans

Beans are a good source of proteins that every runner requires them fit, strong and rejuvenated for the coming competition that they are about to take part in. in addition to this, they are a cheap source of iron since beans are considered be the very few pants that can supply iron that is required by the human body. Iron is important for the functioning and the formation of the red blood cells some important blood component responsible for the circulation oxygen in the blood.

As an athlete runs, the amount of oxygen he requires doubles because a lot of carbohydrates are continuously being converted to energy through the metabolism which requires this oxygen. An athlete who lacks iron will thus have an insufficient supply of oxygen in the blood stream rendering him or her weakness for the exercise.

Beans are also a source of fats I low amounts, something that every athlete requires to remain healthy and fit.

How To Incorporate In The Diet

Beans have been used many times with soup and stews. But one perfect example where one can get the simplest meal is taking rice and beans. The rice will be the chief supplier of the carbs that will be store of energy while the beans will perform the specific roles described above.

Ingredients

- 1 labeled package of rice

- 1 package of orzo

- 1 glass of yoghurt

- ½ glass of honey (creamy Dijon salad)

- ¼ glass of milk

- ¼ glass of honey (mustard Dijon)

- 1/3 glass of parmesan cheese (grated)

- 15 oz. can of black beans that is rinsed and drained

- 12 oz. white chicken

- 3 chopped bell peppers

- 1 tomato

Preparative Procedure

Begin by cooking the rice as stipulated in the package. Cook the orzo as well as described. As that continues mix the yoghurt, the salad dressing, the milk, the lemon juice, the cheese and the milk. After that you can then add the salt together with the pepper. To the resultant mixture, add the chicken, the beans, the peppers, the tomatoes, the wild rice and the orzo and mix them well. Put the mixture in the fridge for 2 hours then serve.

4. Salmon

Salmon being a fish is an excellent source of proteins that every runner needs to replenish the muscle tissues that are used up when running. In addition to this basic importance, the salmon fish is also an important source of omega 3 fats. Omega 3 fats are responsible for the brain functioning. It is also an important nutrient that prevents one from having a heart complication and even the high blood pressure condition. By taking this fish species, the runner can get vitamins type A and B. minerals that the body requires are also other benefits that come from taking the fish.

How To Incorporate In The Diet

With salmon, you can take it with any other meal making it very versatile. You can bake it, grill it and even poach it. The choice depends on the best mode that suits a runner.

A runner can also choose to have the canned salmon.

Ingredients

- 14 oz. salmon

- 16 oz. black beans

- 1 glass of green salsa

- About 1 glass of cheese (Muenster)

- 2 avocados

- 1 glass of grape tomatoes

- 8 shells of taco

- Toppings of taco

Preparation Procedures

Mix all the ingredients above leaving aside the taco shells. Heat the taco shells by following the procedures on the package. Then arrange the salmon tacos with the ingredients before serving.

5. Sweet Potatoes

Sweet potatoes like most other types of food fit for runner are a good source of natural carbohydrates. By ingesting them, the runner can get vitamin A from these potatoes which are the best type of an antioxidant that the body requires. In addition to the supplements above, sweet potatoes are an excellent source of vitamin C. The mineral content that one can get from the food are iron and potassium.

How to Incorporate In the Diet

Generally sweet potatoes are basically tasty naturally since they are sweetened by Mother Nature. Their mode of cooking represents a rather simplified way where one does not need a lot of things to make a meal out of it. Everything is simple and tasty with sweet potatoes.

Cooking them is a rather simple procedure where one can use the microwave for cooking, and then you can choose to add either butter or margarine to make them tastier. Another procedure that one can follow is to cut them into slices and bake them to get some fries.

Sweet Potato Casserole Recipe

Ingredients

- 2.5 pounds of cut and peeled sweet potatoes

- 3.25 glass of sugar (brown)

- ¼ glass of softened butter

- 1.5 teaspoons of salt

- ½ teaspoon of vanilla extract

- ½ glass of chopped pecans

Preparation Procedures

Heat the oven to high temperatures. Put the sweet potato in an oven and cover them with cold water then boil. Reduce the heat then drain. Put them in a bowl then add sugar together with the rest of the 3 ingredients then you mash the mixture then fold the pecans and bake till they turn golden.

6. Yogurt With Low Fat

If you are looking for a liquid food supplement that will keep you nourished as a runner then the yoghurt named above is the perfect choice for you. Having the low fat content ensures that the runner is safe from any form of physical unfitness when exercising. Since milk is an excellent source of protein then you will get the chance to get all the proteins that comes from the yoghurt. Additionally, you will get the calcium minerals that are essential for bone formation, and keeping you safe from stress fractures.

How To Incorporate In The Diet

You can opt to consume the low fat yoghurt as a snack since they come in containers. This can be done either in the mid-morning or even in the mid afternoon. If you are a bit creative or you want to try something new then you can make smoothies using the yoghurt itself with some frozen fruits.

Ingredients

- About 1 glass of strawberries (frozen)

- 1 glass of pineapple chunk (frozen but unsweetened)

- 1 glass of vanilla soy milk

- 2 teaspoonful of honey

- ½ glass of yoghurt (vanilla soy)

Preparatory Procedure

Put the strawberries together with the pineapple in the blender then add the rest of the ingredients and cover them before stirring till it gets smooth.

7. Bananas

When running, you lose a large amount of minerals through sweating. One of the mineral that one loses pretty fast is potassium. This mineral is particularly important for the contraction of muscles as they protect them from cramping. Most of the athletes consider bananas as the best food to take as they rarely cause any form of stomach issues. This explains why most of them take it before running. Bananas are good source of potassium as well as carbohydrates.

How To Incorporate In The Diet

One can take a ripe banana as a snack or even as a part of a meal. They are very convenient because of the form in which they come in. you can choose to make a smoothie out of it by combining it with milk. Or you could just add bananas to cereal.

Ingredients

- 2 bananas

- 1 glass of pineapple chunks (frozen but unsweetened)

- 1 glass of ice

- About a glass of pineapple juice (unsweetened)

- 1 glass of banana yoghurt

- Cinnamon

Preparation Procedures

Put the bananas, the pineapple together with the ice in a blender then pour the pineapple juice into the mixture and add the yoghurt on top. Cover the mixture and pound until they are smooth then add the cinnamon to garnish before serving 3.

8. Peanut Butter

There are those runners who run not to compete but to lose weight. The peanut butter experience gives them a chance to eat something that is not only tasty but is also satisfying making it the best food for such people. With a high amount of fiber, one can be sure to be full for most part of the day when taking it and you will never increase in weight unless you eat more than the required amount. Peanut butter is also an excellent source of proteins that every runner needs to repair the damaged tissues and get the muscles replenished.

The peanut butter is also an excellent source of fats that are healthy to consume. They also have very low amounts of cholesterols.

How To Incorporate In The Diet

One can take the peanut butter on whole grain. You can also choose to take it with bread for breakfast.

Peanut Butter, Banana With Chia Seed Recipe

Ingredients

• 1 toasted bagel

• 2 teaspoons of peanut butter

• 1 sliced banana

• ½ teaspoons of chia seeds

Preparation Procedures

On each slice of the toasted bagel, spread the peanut butter. Then add the

9. Carrots

Every runner requires a good immune system. For you to get the best immunity, then you need to take foods that are rich in vitamins. Carrots are the perfect examples of such foods. They offer the vitamin A to boost the immune system. If you are a runner who is very sensitive in as much your weight is concerned, then this is the perfect food that you should take since it helps you fill up very first. They are also very low on the amount of calories they deliver when taken. Vitamin A is also a food supplement that is important improved vision.

How To Incorporate In The Diet

You can eat carrots before dinner as they will quench your hunger for food giving you the advantage of not over eating during dinner.

Ingredients

- ¾ glass of fresh pineapples cut into pieces

- ½ glass of ice

- ¼ glass of orange juice

- ¼ glass of carrots cut into pieces

- ½ banana

Preparation Procedures

Place all the ingredients in a blender. Then blend then until they turn smooth and frothy.

10. Quinoa

This easy to cook food is an alternative to other foods above, especially for runners who would love to change their diet. This type of tasty food is not only rich in protein but is rich in carbohydrate as well. From it one can derive little amounts of fat that is healthy.

How To Incorporate In The Diet

Since it is very easy to cook this type of food, then you can always have it as a meal in combination with other meals.

You can have this type of food with chicken or even fish. You can choose to take it with salads.

Ingredients

- ½ of lemon

- 4 fish fillets

- 2 teaspoons of olive oil

- 30g of butter

- 150g of macro Quinoa

- 1 zucchini chopped

- 1 onion red in color

- 1 garlic clove

- 375 ml of chicken stalk

- 50g of half dried tomatoes chopped

- 2 tablespoons of toasted pine nuts

Preparation Procedure

Cut the lemon into strips. Add salt and pepper to the fish. Heat the oil and cook then until they become light brown in color by lowering the temperature, cook the remaining ingredients i.e. Quinoa, onion, garlic and zucchini then stir for about 12 minutes. Reduce the heat then place the fish on top of the Quinoa mixture and add any juice that is available. A fork can be used to fluff the Quinoa before serving and toping up with dried tomato, lemon rind and pine nuts.